I0439773

Masturbation Addiction

The Ultimate Guide for How to Overcome This Time-Consuming Addiction

presentation of the information is without contract or any type of guarantee assurance.

The trademarks that are used are without any consent, and the publication of the trademark is without permission or backing by the trademark owner. All trademarks and brands within this book are for clarifying purposes only and are the owned by the owners themselves, not affiliated with this document.

Table Of Contents

Introduction

First off, I really want to thank you for downloading this book. The pages in this book were developed through years of experiences that I have gone through, as well as what has proven to work for others I have talked to and have researched. I also want to congratulate you for taking the time to understand your own masturbation addiction and how you can overcome it.

I can guarantee that you will find this book useful if you make sure to implement what you learn in the following pages. The important thing is that you IMPLEMENT what you learn. A masturbation addiction is not conquered overnight but the important thing to remember is that it is definitely possible for you to overcome it. What I am giving you is the information so that you can understand your own mind, how masturbation addictions negatively affect you, as well as the steps you will need to make that journey.

Many people experience an addiction to masturbation and aren't really aware of the what is provoking it. There is a difference between casual masturbation one to three times a week and chronically masturbating. As you go through these pages, you'll get a better understanding of what masturbation addiction really is, the research that has been done on masturbation addiction, and you will learn several ways that you can overcome it. We will dive into what is going on in your mind, how your body reacts to your triggers, how your free time can influence the habits you develop, as well as what work is required of you to get past the roadblocks you have.

I recommend that you take notes while you are reading this short ebook. This will ensure that you get the most out of the information in here. I want you to feel that you made a purchase that is worth your money and I want you to look over the notes of this book even after you've finished reading it. The notes will help you to pinpoint exactly what you need to implement, and by writing things down, you will be able to recall specifics and how to handle certain situations when they arise.

Lastly, remember that everything in this book has been compiled through research, my own experiences, as well as the experiences of others, so feel free to question what you have read in this book. I encourage you to do your own research on the things that you want to look deeper into. The more you understand about your own mind and body, the better off you'll be. To overcome a masturbation addiction, it will take some work on your part but you can do it! So remember to read with confidence and an open   mind!

Chapter 1:

Masturbation In Our Everyday Lives

If you belong to the 40% of males or 22% of females who admit to masturbating daily, then you could be one of the 797,151 Americans who are masturbating at this very moment. If you started masturbating since you were twelve years old, by the time you are 28 and are ready to get married, you would have probably wasted 1,081 hours playing with your thing.

Onan and His Sin

Masturbation has always been inextricably attributed to Onan, a biblical character who has been the etymological cause for the word onanism—a synonym for masturbation. Onan committed the sin of "wasting his seed (semen) on the ground."

However, the story of Onan has been viewed differently, focusing on and establishing the basis of his error upon the act of masturbation, thereby becoming the primary biblical reference for the religious stigma against it. During coitus, in response to God's and Onan's father's (Judah) request for him to carry out his duty to Tamar as a brother-in-law by fathering her a child, Onan deliberately wasted his semen on the ground, which infuriated God. Due to the prevalent misconception that Onan's masturbation was the cause of God's fury, masturbation has always been strongly prohibited by most religious institutions.

Masturbation and Religion

There is no direct passage from the Bible which condemns masturbation. However, most religious institutions today hold a strong disapproval against sexual activities, including masturbation, that are being performed for reasons other than the very purpose of procreation, and hints about the self-gratifying effect it brings to the participant of those activities. The notion is that it is a manifestation of a selfish desire other than the desire to prioritize the will of the deity for which the particular religion is worshiping.

Some religions consider it a form of uncleanliness that creates mentally corrupting habits and attitudes. Modern views from the members of Christianity, however, are beginning to differ as more and more members are realizing that there is no direct Bible passage that prohibits this act. Strong religious prohibition against the act remains though, in religions that consider chastity and celibacy as the basis for the ideal lifestyle.

Addiction

The pleasure derived from masturbation caused by the production of neurotransmitters and hormones such as acetylcholine, dopamine and serotonin, is a powerful factor in sexual conditioning, which is, consequently, the primary cause of masturbation addiction. Sexual conditioning, like any forms of conditioning, can be summarized as "a process in which a behavior is encouraged through a reward (pleasure)."

The three requirements for addiction are:

The act should be easy. The processes that lead to addiction are usually those which can easily be replicated and performed. It should not, as much as possible, cost anything and can be performed anytime and anywhere.

It should make you feel good. Unless an action gives you a pleasurable feeling, why would you want to continue it? Almost all forms of addiction have roots that can be traced back to pleasure "in the moment".

You should want to experience it again. The last requirement for addiction is the desire for re-experience. The uncontrollable desire to experience the pleasure you experienced at the same or at greater degree, is the "loop" part in masturbation addiction. As long as you want to experience pleasure, you will find ways to attain it.

Chemical Basis for Addiction

These three requirements are met by masturbation. It is also noteworthy to point out that the chemicals produced by the brain before, during and after orgasm have similar effects as drugs such as marijuana and tobacco, in such a way that it alters the perception of the brain. Addiction to masturbation is believed to be attributed to two factors:

Sensitization

Recurrent pleasurable feelings caused by regular masturbation encourages the growth of the synapses in the pleasure centers within the brain, which cause an increased perception of pleasure in a process called sensitization. These areas, which form what is called the "reward circuit", reinforce a person's desire to masturbate again.

Desensitization

On the other hand, over-exposure to these neurotransmitters and hormones renders the brain incapable of feeling the same level of pleasure again—a process called desensitization. This causes frustration on the part of the person masturbating, which encourages him/her to perform the act once more in the hope of achieving this preconceived notion of pleasure.

Prevalence

Entrepreneurs have exploited the potential that can be harnessed from masturbation as being a widespread phenomenon. In fact, it has become a lucrative industry and is the cause of over 2.5 million sales in the fleshlight (a type of toy used for masturbating).

New studies reveal that 92% of women ages 18-30 masturbate regularly. The study is based upon the results from interviews with 1,000 women, of which, 9 out of 10 admitted to having masturbated at an average of about three times a week.

Chapter 2:

Common Myths About Masturbation

In the hopes of regulating masturbation to conform to societal norms and religious doctrines prohibiting the act, people have invented stories about the superficial dangers of masturbation.

Masturbation causes blindness.

There is no direct evidence that correlates masturbation to the impairment of eyesight. How can a mechanism that happens down below affect something that is up above?

Fact:

Excessive masturbation, however, can aggravate eye floaters, says one study. Eye floaters are squiggly lines, rod-like bacteria or amoeboid projections, that distort a person's vision. Experts believe that eye floaters, which are, in itself, not a disease, is a sign of serious eye problems.

During masturbation, the brain produces acetylcholine. A depletion of which could lead to the depletion of a phytochemical in the rod visual sensory nerves, which result in eye floaters. Excessive masturbation causes a greater degree of depletion, which further aggravates eye floaters.

Masturbation can damage the genitals.

Over the course of many years of evolution, human genitals have become tough and are able to withstand damage due to sexual activity and even masturbation.

Fact:

Under prolonged use, however, and without proper lubrication, the tender skin of the male genitals is susceptible to chafing. It is advised, therefore, that a suitable lubricant, preferably one that is water-based, must be used prior to masturbation to avoid this.

Masturbation causes mental illness.

There is no direct evidence that points to a link between mental illness and masturbation. As a matter of fact, experts have been recommending masturbation as a way to relieve sexual tension and anxiety.

Fact:

The release of neurotransmitters such as dopamine and serotonin before, during and after orgasm is enough to relieve a person from stress, depression and anxiety. This signifies that masturbation, on the contrary, is a viable remedy to the precursors of mental illness, rather than the cause of it.

Masturbation is sexually exhaustive.

Another myth regarding masturbation is that it depletes a person's vitality since the sexual fluids are said to contain the very essence of life itself. Our body, however, is capable of producing sexual fluids soon after a person has expelled some. This process has also been observed to have never drained a person of vitality, although the relaxing effect after an orgasm tends to make a person look exhausted.

Fact:
The seminal fluid in males is constantly being created and produced by the prostate gland in as much as the testicles are able to create sperm, the moment after the reserves of the sperm are depleted. Although the creation of this fluid uses up resources of the body such as the mineral zinc, the presence of the said mineral in the diet replenishes what is used.

Chapter 3:

Advantages and Disadvantages of Masturbation

Aside from being intellectual and emotional creatures, humans by nature are sexual beings, too. Nature has placed a desire for man and woman to seek sexual pleasure to encourage procreation and survival. With this, nature has provided an elaborate and efficient tool — the reproductive system — which is designed to aid humans in proliferating while enjoying the pleasures brought about by sexual activity.

Although there are no known effects for the disuse of human sexual parts, proper use of it, however, brings about a class of benefits, while the misuse or overuse of it causes a multitude of undesirable consequences.

Advantages

Here are the benefits of masturbation:

It provides an alternative to intercourse.

The UK Government, along with other European nations are beginning to understand the positive effects of encouraging masturbation among teens in curbing the rate of teenage pregnancy. They believe that the underlying factor in the commission of premarital sex among teens is their desire to attain sexual gratification — something that can also be achieved through masturbation. In their slogan "an orgasm a day keeps the doctor away," these nations have expressed their resolve to provide an alternative to intercourse — that which does not result in unwanted pregnancy.

It is a means to release sexual tension.

Sexual tension, when not managed effectively, leads to both personal and social difficulties. Sexual tension occurs when an individual has sexual feelings towards another but is not readily consummated, if at all. When not managed, sexual tension could be self-destructive, as it results in depression and decreased self-esteem.

It can also lead to a person to defying moral rules set by the society, as it can propel an individual to find ways to consummate the sexual desire in whatever way possible — socially acceptable or not. Fortunately, masturbation is the best way to release sexual tension other than consummation itself. A person can experience the same sexual gratification as actual sexual contact with the desired person, through masturbation. With the skillful use of the faculty of imagination, one can effectively manage sexual tension.

It is a form of exercise.

Data reveals that inactivity is the leading cause of cardiovascular-related diseases and disabilities, which accounts for 2 million deaths per annum as provided by the World Health Organization. Masturbation is a form of, not only physical but also, mental exercise, which keeps our heart rate, blood pressure and brain chemistry in very good shape.

Increases fertility.

Although excessive masturbation can do more harm than good to fertility, regular masturbation, done at an interval of three or more days, increases fertility in males. This is because masturbation flushes out old sperm, which may have low motility, and replaces them with new sperm cells, which are active and are more capable of surviving the insides of the womb and fertilizing the ovum.

Disadvantages

Over-doing masturbation has its disadvantages, too. Here are the downsides of masturbation:

Guilty feeling.

Most people, especially those who are bound by strict social and moral rules that look down upon masturbation, suffer from a feeling of shame and guilt. Part of the reason is that most religious institutions consider imagining a person naked, or being in sexual activity with them — a vital component of masturbation — as adulterous.

Bruising or soreness of the genital organs.

Without proper lubrication, those who are circumcised (or had their foreskin removed) may experience soreness or bruising of their venereal organs because of the undue strain caused by over-doing masturbation. When coupled with poor hygiene and dirty hands, bruising and soreness may progress towards infection.

Addictive.

Because masturbation produces elation and intense pleasure brought about by orgasm, it is one of the habits that is difficult to break. Most adolescents resort to masturbation whenever they have some free time. This could lead to their having no time for other aspects of their lives as to the development of their talents and skills.

Causes sex related difficulties.

Masturbation has been observed to cause premature ejaculation among men, in which a man may achieve ejaculation within a few seconds or minutes of penetrating a woman. This causes frustration not only on the part of the man, in which sexual satisfaction is achieved through prolonged and meaningful sexual contact, but also on the part of the woman.

Chapter 4:

How to Overcome Masturbation Addiction

To lead a happy and healthy sexual life it is advised for those who are not regularly having coitus to perform masturbation one to three times a week. Beyond this though, the act is already considered compulsive and addictive and needs to be mitigated. Here are proven steps to help you overcome masturbation addiction:

Make up your mind. Be firm in your resolve to overcome addiction.

Understand your reason for quitting. Remind yourself of the reasons why you would like to overcome your addiction. Whether it is religious, a moral issue, or a personal reason, whatever it is, you have to convince yourself that you will endeavor to overcome your addiction.

The key here is that everyone has their own reasons for overcoming their masturbation addiction. Maybe you are having problems in your relationships, maybe you are religious, or maybe you want to be more productive with your time. It is not anyone else's job to tell you if masturbation is wrong or right. You must decide to commit to this for yourself and stick to your commitment.

Accept the sacrifices.

From time to time, you will be tempted to masturbate. The key concept here is "self-control." By not giving in to the compulsion and by trying to take control, you will gradually overcome this addiction.

Remind yourself of the price at stake. Freedom. Remind yourself that at the end of this detachment process, you will gain control of yourself and this addiction. By doing this, you will get your energy levels up high again and be motivated to continue the process.

Avoid things that sexually arouse you.

Anything that produces sexual tension or arouses you sexually will eventually tempt you to masturbate. Some may think that by exposing themselves to these things, they become better at self-control. What they do not understand, however, is that sexual tension piles up and eventually overwhelms a person.

Do not try to trick yourself by thinking you will just block out all the things that sexually arouse you. To make a lasting change, you must consciously try to avoid situations where your will-power will be low.

Keep your old pornographic materials away from you.

Avoid pornographic sites in the internet. Whenever you are tempted, divert your attention to another activity that brings you pleasure. By doing this, you can release the same chemicals in the brain, but without having to go through the act of masturbating. Realize that if these materials have successfully made your masturbation experience beyond great, then giving you access to them once more will remind you of that feeling, and could potentially turn you on.

Limit your time in the shower.

If you are the type of person who tends to masturbate in the shower or while taking a shower, avoid this temptation by limiting your time spent in the shower. Have a definite plan on how to clean yourself by sequence and stick to your plan. Over time, you will gradually see that the new "shower plan" is turning into a habit and that the old habit is being replaced little by little.

Spend less time being alone.

If you observe that you tend to masturbate whenever nobody is around, then avoid occasions where you could be alone. Invite friends over — friends who have similar interests as you. Do solitary activities outside of your room whenever you can. Watch a movie or have a dinner with friends or members of your family. Talk to your brother, sister, or your parents.

Anything that will limit your time being alone will definitely help you achieve this goal. The majority of chronic masturbators have too much free time. With so much free time, they run out of things to do and often times browse their favorite pornographic websites out of boredom.

Think of your future self.

A great technique that has helped many people overcome their masturbation addiction is to think of what their future self would be proud of. Every time you are tempted to masturbate (or any time-wasting activity for that matter), think about yourself in 5, 10, or 20 years from now. What will you be proud that you spent your time doing? Would that 30 minutes be better spent masturbating or going to the gym, studying for your next test, or even calling up an old friend?

By keeping this perspective, you will avoid doing things that aren't going to build your future and, in turn, you will be more aware of your activities throughout the day. Keeping yourself busy with worthwhile things does not only keep you from masturbating. It also helps you discover and develop your potential and uplift your chances for a better life ahead.

Do something creative.

Find a hobby, anything that pleases you and gives you a way to express your skills and talents. If you like music, compose a song, practice an instrument, or simply sing. It is well-known that many artists throughout the centuries have learned to channel their sexual energy into making amazing pieces of art. By learning how to channel that built up energy within you, you can have more productive outlets based on your own interests.

Do something engaging.

Anything that requires your immersion and concentration will be helpful. Read a book or learn a new skill. Reading a book (and finishing it) is particularly helpful not only because it directs your mood and thinking but because it also takes sexual images out of your mind and immerses you in a different mindset all together.

Join clubs and organizations.

If you find yourself having too much spare time (especially if you are still in school), you can join a club, a sports team, or an organization. It will not only divert your attention from masturbation, it will also provide you with a means to make your time worthwhile and will allow you to develop a particular skill and great friendships with other people. Creating friendships in real life has been proven to be more beneficial to our health than by communicating strictly online by chatting.

Perform a physical exercise.

Whenever you feel the need to masturbate or a sexually arousing image enters your mind, make it a point to perform a physical exercise. Either you jog in place, do push-ups and sit-ups, or perform a full course of exercise. Doing a physical exercise will help you take away your thought from masturbating and will exhaust your physical energy, leaving you too tired to masturbate.

Promise yourself a reward.

To further encourage yourself to stay on track, promise yourself something. It could be a video game day or a movie marathon with friends, or you can treat yourself to your favorite food. You need to remind yourself that if you achieve your goal, you will be allowed to celebrate.

Withdraw gradually.

Like any other forms of addiction, there may be withdrawal symptoms, either physiological or psychological. The key is to gradually withdraw from the addiction rather than stopping altogether. Go from twice a day, to once a day, to every other day, to two times a week, to only once a week.

This is a very effective method that people have used and it has proven to be one of the best programs. Remember to have a log where you write down the time of day and what instigated you to masturbate. This is important because you don't want to try to memorize the frequency, as it will be too hard to see the progress you have been making over time.

Give in occasionally.

Realize that your body has been accustomed to releasing sexual tension and is unable to handle sexual tension without immediate release anymore. If you failed to follow the above indicated steps and have a buildup of sexual tension, masturbate to release it. Hence, you will feel exhausted of the withdrawal and will eventually decide to not stop.

Chapter 5:

Life After Masturbation Addiction

Recovery from the addiction to masturbation is not permanent. Over time, exposure to the same triggers or environmental factors that caused the addiction in the first place will cause its reoccurrence. Even after getting over the initial hump, there will still be challenges that must be dealt with.

Sexual tension buildup is inevitable. Evolution has made humans to be sexually active, in order to encourage procreation and reproduction. Humans have a highly-developed sexual component that is easily aroused. Exposure to factors that cause arousal, say visual stimuli for males and emotional and auditory stimuli for females, can cause the buildup of coital tension. It is natural to give in to the temptation once in a while and perform masturbation. After all, occasional masturbation has its advantages, too.

Tolerance to anxiety and stress will change. Having neurotransmitters like serotonin, acetylcholine and dopamine in the bloodstream fulfills a requirement for personal satisfaction that eventually leads to a sense of well-being. Stopping frequent masturbation will cause a significant decrease in the production of these chemicals in the body, so it is imperative that you find other ways to manage stress and anxiety in order to break free from the dependence on these chemicals for relief.

Emotional and sexual response will increase. You will realize, too, that your emotional and sexual acuity have increased after a prolonged period of abstinence from masturbation. Instead of entertaining its negative impact upon your life, use it to your advantage. Fall in love with a person and devote your emotional energy to him or her rather than divide your attention to many persons.

Most people who are content with their lives are those who have found alternative ways to manage their urges and have found other means to find joy in life. There are many opportunities for, and sources of gratification other than, what are sexual and physical. Finding these alternatives will greatly improve your quality of life and your sense of well-being — that which is free from the grasp of the addiction to masturbation.

One of the biggest keys to developing a healthier relationship with your masturbation habits is to remember that the best way to overcome your addiction is to substitute your time with other fulfilling activities: that is the over-arching theme of this book. I dare you to fill your life with joyous, fulfilling, and energy filled activities while masturbating three times a day. It is just not likely to happen. We each have only so much built-up energy each day and we all have 24 hours in a day. How we decide to spend those hours and that energy is up to us. **This is the key for you to remember in order for you to make the change.**

Conclusion

I worked hard on creating the best guide for "overcoming a masturbation addiction" that I could. These are all the strategies and information that have worked for me, as well as others that I have talked to and researched. I guarantee if you stay consistent they will work for you as well. Be optimistic about your current situation and make small progress each day!

If you feel like you learned something from this book, please take the time to share your thoughts with me by sending me a message! I would also appreciate it if you left a review on Amazon.

Thank you and good luck in your journey!